AF680698

# Almost

## A Memoir for Anyone Who Felt Counted Out, Left Behind, Or Written Off – And Kept Going Anyway

Tiffanii Smith, MD

Copyright © 2024 Tiffanii Smith, MD

All rights reserved. No part of this publication may be reproduced, distributed, or transmitted in any form or by any means, including photocopying, recording, or other electronic or mechanical methods, without the prior written permission of the author, except in the case of brief quotations embodied in critical reviews and certain other noncommercial uses permitted by copyright law.

ISBN: 979-8-90271-042-4

# DEDICATION

To my firstborn son, Deshon—
my greatest supporter and my steady ground.

When I question myself, you are the voice that reminds me who I am.

Your belief in me has carried me through moments of doubt and into purpose.

This book exists because you stood beside me, lifted me, and never let me forget my worth.

All that I am, and all that I continue to become, is strengthened by you.

# PREFACE

There were so many moments in my life when the story could have ended differently.

Moments when walking away would have made sense. Moments when giving up felt more logical than trying again. Moments when I stood so close to the edge that I didn't know if I was stepping forward—or falling.

I didn't grow up planning to be strong.
I grew up learning how to survive.

I made decisions at a young age that forced me into adulthood before I was ready for it. Decisions that came from fear, confusion, and wanting to be loved more than I wanted to be safe. Those choices left me carrying labels I never imagined I would wear—high school dropout, homeless, teenage mother. I didn't choose those names for myself. Life handed them to me, and for a long time, I didn't know how to hand them back.

Before I had time to dream, I had to endure.
Before I had time to plan, I had to survive.

As the years passed, the struggle didn't disappear—it just changed shape. I found myself in a marriage that hurt more than it healed. In jobs that barely paid the bills. In a life that looked full on the outside but felt empty on the inside. I became a mother of three while still trying to figure out how to become a woman myself.

I wanted better—but I didn't yet know how to reach it. Some days, I didn't even know if I deserved it.

There were seasons when I almost stayed stuck. Almost accepted that this was as good as life would ever get. Almost believed the quiet lie that said, *This is all you are. This is all you'll ever be.* I came closer than I ever admitted to folding under the weight of everything I carried.

But somehow, I didn't.

Not because I felt strong.
Not because I had a plan.
Not because I was fearless.

I kept going because stopping felt worse than trying one more time.

There were nights I sat alone, wondering how my life had become something I barely recognized. Nights when I replayed every mistake, every wrong turn, every moment I wished I could undo. Nights when I looked at my children sleeping and asked myself if I was enough for them—if I was giving them the life they deserved, or just the best I could manage with what I had left.

I doubted myself more times than I can count.
I doubted my choices.
I doubted my worth.

And still, I stayed.

I learned something along the way that no one teaches you when you're young—willpower isn't loud. It doesn't always feel like courage. Sometimes it shows up quietly, barely holding together, whispering just enough strength to get you through the next hour.

People say, *Where there's a will, there's a way.*
What they don't tell you is that sometimes your will is exhausted, scared, and unsure—but it still counts.

Because even the smallest will can create a way when the alternative is giving up.

This book is not the story of someone who always believed she would make it.
It is the story of someone who almost didn't.

Almost gave up.
Almost stayed broken.
Almost stopped dreaming.
Almost believed the pain would get the final word.

But didn't.

If you are reading this and you feel like you are standing in your own *almost*—almost done, almost defeated, almost too tired to keep trying—I wrote this for you. Not as a lecture. Not as a formula for success. But as proof that even when you are unsure how to win, you can still survive. And sometimes survival is the first brave step toward becoming something you never thought you could be.

This is not a story about being unstoppable.
It is a story about being **almost lost—and still here.**

And if that is where you are right now...
You are not finished yet.

# Table of Contents

# HIGH SCHOOL

I didn't grow up thinking my life would be hard. Hard just became normal.

Some people can point to one moment when everything went wrong. I can't. For me, it was a slow unraveling—a series of quiet disappointments, missed guidance, and wrong turns that added up before I realized what was happening. By the time I understood I was in trouble, I was already deep in it.

There were so many paths my life could have taken. I could have accepted homelessness as my fate. I could have settled into the idea that being a teenage mother was all I would ever be. I could have believed that dropping out of high school meant I had dropped out of life. I could have worn the label of a battered woman and never imagined myself as anything else.

I almost did.

There were days when survival felt like the only dream I was allowed to have. A roof. A meal. One quiet night without fear. Wanting more felt selfish when I was barely holding on to what I had.

And yet—even then—I never fully fit into the life I was living. It was like wearing someone else's coat: heavy, uncomfortable, never quite mine. Something in me kept whispering that this wasn't the end of my story. I didn't know what my future looked like. I just knew I wasn't meant to stay where I was.

Growing up without my mother left a space in me that I didn't have words for back then. My father did everything he could to raise four children on his own. We weren't rich, but we were cared for. We had lights. We had food. We had stability—at least on the surface. But there are needs that go deeper than shelter. There are questions only a mother can answer. Wounds only a mother can see.

Without that guidance, I learned about life from the people closest to me. My sister became my model for womanhood. What she did, I wanted to do. What she wore, I wanted to wear. I didn't know I was following footsteps that would lead me into situations I wasn't ready to face.

By twelve years old, I was already searching for love in the wrong places.

What began as innocent phone calls turned into a relationship that slowly changed the way I saw myself. I didn't recognize danger when it first appeared. I recognized attention. I recognized feeling wanted. And when fear finally showed its face, I didn't call it abuse. I called it love.

That misunderstanding almost cost me everything.

By high school, my world had become chaotic. I skipped classes. I drifted away from the things that once grounded me—sports, structure, dreams. I followed a boy whose reputation I ignored because being loved felt better than being safe. I told myself I could handle it. I told myself it wasn't that bad.

But it was.

The abuse didn't start loudly. It never does. It started quietly—with words that cut deeper than fists. Then came the pushing. Then the choking. Then the fear that settled in my bones and made me believe I couldn't leave even if I wanted to.

I almost accepted that this was what love looked like.

I hid everything. I didn't tell my father. I didn't tell my brothers. I protected the person who was hurting me because I didn't want him hurt in return. That's the strange thing about pain—it can twist your loyalty until you start defending the very thing that's destroying you.

By sixteen, I was exhausted in ways no teenager should be. By seventeen, I was pregnant.

The day I found out felt like the world stopped spinning. I was still trying to survive my own life—now I was responsible for another. I was scared of telling my father. Scared of disappointing him. Scared of admitting how far I had drifted from the girl he raised.

I thought about running.
And then I did.

I left home without saying goodbye. I didn't even have the courage to explain. I just disappeared—too afraid to face the consequences of my own choices. Looking back now, I understand how cruel that must have been. I was trying to escape my fear, but I created someone else's.

That was the moment I became almost everything I never wanted to be:
almost alone,
almost homeless,
almost broken beyond repair.

But it was also the moment that forced me to grow.

I didn't know it then, but that scared teenage girl was standing at the edge of the life she would one day fight to rise above. She didn't have a plan. She didn't have confidence. She didn't even have a home.

All she had was a choice she barely understood yet—to keep going, even when everything in her wanted to stop.

# PREGNANCY

## *Almost*

Pregnancy didn't feel real at first. It felt like something that had happened to someone else—some other girl who had her life together, who knew what she was doing, who had a plan. Not me. I was still trying to figure out where I would sleep next, how I would survive the next argument, the next threat, the next day.

I was seventeen years old and already tired in a way that sleep couldn't fix.

People had opinions. Some whispered that I should end it—end the pregnancy, end the problem, end the embarrassment. Others warned me that having a child would ruin my life. And maybe they were right in their own way. But something in me couldn't let go. I didn't feel brave. I felt scared. I didn't feel strong. I felt trapped. But I chose to keep the baby anyway—not because I was confident, but because I couldn't live with the idea of erasing a life when I was still fighting to save my own.

That decision pushed me straight into the unknown.

I left home without telling my father. No explanation. No goodbye. Just fear carrying me out the door. I stayed with my boyfriend's family, pretending I was okay while quietly breaking inside. I didn't understand then how deeply that must have hurt my father—to come home and find his child gone, with no idea where she was or if she was safe. I only understood my own terror. I only knew how to run.

Homelessness doesn't always look like sleeping on the street. Sometimes it looks like sleeping on couches, staying where you're allowed to stay—until you're not. Sometimes it looks like being a guest everywhere and belonging nowhere.

That was my life.

I drifted from place to place while my body changed and my fear grew. And still, the abuse didn't stop. Even pregnant, I was pushed, slapped, and choked. I told myself it wouldn't happen again. I told myself he was sorry. I told myself love was supposed to hurt sometimes.

I almost believed that lie.

There were moments when I thought the baby inside me would be the thing that changed everything. That becoming a mother would soften him. That he would grow up because I had to. But life doesn't change just because you hope it will.

One day, after another violent episode, I sat crying in my sister's apartment—my body bruised, my heart exhausted, my future uncertain. I had nowhere to go. No money. No plan. Just a baby growing inside me and fear growing beside it.

For the first time, I wasn't just afraid for myself anymore.
I was afraid for my child.

And still, I stayed.

That's what people don't understand about abuse—you don't stay because you don't see the danger. You stay because the danger becomes familiar. And familiarity can feel safer than the unknown.

By the time my boyfriend went back to jail, I was pregnant, homeless, and completely alone. His parents took me in, and for the first time in a long time, I felt something I hadn't felt in years—stability. Not comfort. Not security. Just stability. A bed. Meals. A place where no one was hitting me.

I learned what it felt like to breathe again.

His mother didn't have to help me, but she did. She taught me things I didn't know how to ask for—how to care for myself, how to prepare for a baby, how to survive without falling apart every day. I was still young. Still scared. Still unsure. But for the first time in a long time, I wasn't completely alone.

When the day came to give birth, I was barely prepared. I was still a child having a child. But on July 1st, everything changed. I brought my son into the world with no pain medication, no real idea of what I was doing—just instinct, fear, and love colliding in one moment.

He was tiny. Fragile. And mine.

For the first time in my life, I felt something stronger than fear.

Responsibility.

Then came the roses.

I was lying in the hospital bed when I saw them sitting on the table. Red. Bright. Alive. And on the card were two words I never expected to see.

*Love, Dad.*

I cried harder than I had through any beating, any heartbreak, any disappointment. Because I thought I had lost him forever. I thought I had ruined everything. But in that moment, I realized something that would carry me for years to come—love doesn't disappear just because you fall.

That was the first time I understood that I wasn't completely alone in this world.

Motherhood came fast and hard. Sleepless nights. Endless feedings. A baby crying when I didn't know what he needed. I felt useless sometimes. Like I was failing at the one thing that mattered most. But his grandmother showed me patience. She showed me that parenting wasn't about perfection—it was about showing up, even when you didn't know how.

I tried to go back to school. I wanted to finish high school. I wanted to prove to myself—and to my father—that I wasn't done yet. But life had other plans. When I entered a program for teen mothers, I was told I couldn't attend high school anymore. I had to choose between stability and the dream of walking across that stage.

I chose stability.

And that choice broke my heart.

That was the first time I realized how often survival demands sacrifices that dreams aren't ready for.

I moved into a shelter for teen mothers. Twelve of us. Twelve young girls with babies and stories heavy enough to fill rooms. It wasn't the kind of place people imagine when they hear the word "shelter." It looked more like a small motel. But the rules were strict, and the future felt uncertain.

Still, I was grateful.

I learned how to live on almost nothing.
How to stretch food.
How to budget dollars that barely existed.
How to be a mother when I still felt like a child.

Some days I felt proud.
Some days I felt ashamed.
Most days, I felt tired.

But I stayed.

And in that staying, something started to grow—not confidence yet, not courage—but endurance.

I didn't know it then, but I was learning the hardest lesson of my life:
Sometimes the first victory isn't success.
Sometimes it's simply not quitting.

# THE STRIP CLUB

*Almost*

Leaving the shelter felt like freedom on the surface. I had survived the hardest year of my young life. I had learned how to stretch a dollar, how to keep my child fed, how to stand on my own feet even when they shook. I had a roof. I had routines. I had rules. And somehow, rules had started to feel like safety.

But when that year ended, safety disappeared again.

I was still young. Still uneducated. Still carrying a past that followed me into every room. I wanted independence—but independence without support is just another form of fear. I moved into my own place with assistance, finally having a door that locked behind me and a space that was mine. For the first time, I wasn't homeless.

But I was still barely surviving.

I worked when I could. I tried jobs that paid just enough to keep me from falling completely apart. Five dollars an hour. Dead-end shifts. Long days that led nowhere. I stared at computer screens until my eyes burned, pretending this was a step forward when it felt more like standing still.

I told myself it was temporary.
I told myself it was better than nothing.

And then one weekend, I heard about fast money.

It wasn't glamorous at first. It didn't sound dangerous. It just sounded like relief. A way to stop worrying every time my child needed something I couldn't afford. A way to breathe.

They called it dancing.

I called it a chance.

The first time I stepped onto that stage, I didn't feel shame. I felt power. I felt seen. After years of feeling invisible—bruised, forgotten, dismissed—being noticed felt like medicine. The lights were bright. The music was loud. The men looked at me like I mattered.

And for a moment, I believed it.

I told myself it would only be temporary. Just weekends. Just out of town. Just until I saved enough money to get ahead. I didn't see the trap forming around me. I didn't realize how easy it is to get used to fast cash when you've spent your life counting pennies.

I almost convinced myself this was progress.

But the truth is, I wasn't moving forward. I was drifting sideways—into a world that looks glamorous from the outside and feels empty on the inside. Nights turned into mornings. Money turned into spending. Spending turned into nothing saved. And before I knew it, this life had become normal too.

I worked during the night. I slept during the day. My son stayed with his grandmother while I chased survival in neon lights and loud music. I told myself I was doing what I had to do. But deep down, I knew something wasn't right.

I wasn't building a future.
I was escaping the present.

That world was darker than I ever imagined. Drugs everywhere. Violence hiding behind smiles. Girls disappearing. Stories whispered about women who never made it home. I watched people ruin their lives one night at a time and told myself I was different. That I had boundaries. That I would never go that far.

But I was still standing in the same room.

I saw how easy it was to be degraded. How quickly your body becomes a product. How fast dignity gets traded for dollars when you don't believe that you're worth more.

One night, a man waved a single dollar in front of me—just one—while making me parade in front of his family like a joke. He never gave me the money. He just laughed.

And something in me finally broke.

Not loudly.
Not dramatically.
Quietly.

In that moment, I saw myself clearly for the first time in years. Not as strong. Not as empowered. But as someone being reduced to whatever someone else was willing to pay.

I almost stayed.

But I didn't.

I walked out of that club with no savings, no backup plan, and no idea what I would do next. All I knew was that I couldn't keep living like that. I was tired of surviving in ways that were killing me slowly.

Leaving that life didn't magically fix everything. I didn't step into success. I stepped into uncertainty. I took whatever job would hire me. Warehouses. Restaurants. Salons. Anything honest, anything legal, anything that let me come home without feeling ashamed.

I was broke again.
I was tired again.
I was scared again.

But this time, I was free.

I didn't know it then, but this was another turning point. Not a victory—just a narrow escape. One of many moments where my life could have kept spiraling and somehow didn't.

I wasn't unstoppable.
I wasn't strong.
I wasn't fearless.

I was almost lost.

And still, here I was—standing in the middle of my mess, trying one more time to choose a different future.

# MARRIAGE

*Almost*

Leaving that life behind didn't turn everything around. It just brought me back to reality—the kind that doesn't sparkle, doesn't applaud, and doesn't offer shortcuts. I went from fast money to slow days, from late nights to early mornings, from noise to silence. I traded one kind of exhaustion for another.

I took whatever work I could find. Salons. Restaurants. Warehouses. Any place that would let me clock in and prove I was trying to live differently. None of it paid much. None of it felt like purpose. But it felt honest. And after everything I had lived through, honesty felt like progress.

Still, I was tired in ways no paycheck could fix.

I was raising a child while still trying to heal from being one. I was learning how to show up for someone else when

I barely knew how to show up for myself. My son needed stability. I was still learning what that even meant.

And just when I thought life might finally settle down, it shifted again.

I met someone new—not because I was ready, but because I was lonely. I didn't go into it looking for love. I went into it looking for relief. He felt safe. He felt different. He said he would never hurt me. And I wanted so badly to believe that this time would be different.

Then I found out I was pregnant again.

The news didn't bring joy at first. It brought fear. Fear of starting over. Fear of repeating mistakes. Fear of becoming the woman with too many children and not enough answers. I had already survived teenage motherhood once. I didn't know if I had the strength to do it again.

I almost didn't.

But once again, I chose life—not because I felt brave, but because I didn't know how to choose anything else.

Money was tight. So tight that every decision felt like a gamble. I was working, but never catching up. Government assistance filled the gaps that my income couldn't. I hated needing it, but I was grateful for it. Pride doesn't feed children. Survival does.

When my second son was born, I thought the hardest part would be sleepless nights and endless diapers. I was wrong. The hardest part was fear—fear that I would fail him the way I felt I had failed myself.

Then came the diagnosis.

A glimmer in his eye. A specialist visit. Words I didn't understand but felt in my chest like weights. Surgery. Decisions I wasn't prepared to make. I was young. Broke. Uneducated in medical matters. And suddenly, I was responsible for choices that would shape my child's future.

We did the best we could with the information we had. And sometimes, that still isn't enough.

Watching him struggle because of decisions I made as his mother nearly broke me. I carried guilt that no apology could erase. I carried questions that never stopped echoing—*If I had known more, would his life be different? If I had resources, would the outcome have changed?*

Those questions followed me for years.

Life kept moving, even when I felt stuck. I kept working. I kept raising my children. I kept trying to believe that this wasn't where my story ended. But deep down, I still felt like a woman running in place—busy, exhausted, and going nowhere.

Then I got married.

Not because everything was perfect.
Not because we were ready.
But because I was tired of doing life alone.

Marriage didn't save us. It didn't fix our wounds. It only revealed how unhealed we both were. We argued. We struggled financially. We misunderstood each other constantly. I wanted growth. He wanted comfort. I wanted stability. He wanted escape.

And slowly, the love turned into tension.

When our daughter was born, I should have felt complete. Instead, I felt overwhelmed. Postpartum depression wrapped itself around me like a fog I couldn't shake. I stayed in bed. I avoided mirrors. I avoided conversations. I avoided myself.

I almost disappeared inside my own life.

Eventually, I stood up again—because I had to. Not because I felt better, but because my children needed me. I went back to work. I carried on. I smiled when I could. I stayed quiet when I couldn't.

But the marriage kept unraveling.

Arguments turned into resentment. Resentment turned into distance. And one day, distance turned into violence. The man who promised he would never hit me became the man who did.

In that moment, something shifted inside me.

Not fear.
Not sadness.
Resolve.

I had been a battered girl once. I would not be a battered woman again.

That was the day I chose myself—not boldly, not dramatically—but firmly. I left the marriage. I walked away from everything I thought I needed to survive and stood alone again, this time with three children and no safety net.

I worked overnight shifts so I could be present for my kids during the day. I stood on warehouse floors with aching feet and tired eyes, wondering how my life had come to this—and why I still refused to give up.

I wasn't chasing dreams anymore.
I was just trying to survive.

And yet...somewhere in the middle of exhaustion, something new started to grow. Not hope yet. Not vision. Just a quiet question that refused to leave me alone:

*Is this really all my life will ever be?*

I didn't know the answer.
But for the first time, I was brave enough to ask.

# THE CHURCH

*Almost*

By the time I started looking for God, I wasn't searching for religion. I was searching for relief. My life felt like a series of storms that never fully cleared—just different kinds of rain. I had survived abuse. I had survived poverty. I had survived single motherhood. But survival without healing starts to feel like another kind of prison.

I was tired of being strong.
I was tired of pretending I was okay.
I was tired of carrying everything by myself.

So when someone invited me to church, I went—not because I was hopeful, but because I was desperate.

At first, it felt like the answer I had been praying for. A place to belong. A place where broken people were welcome. A place where I could finally lay my burdens down. I didn't come in with expectations. I came in with wounds.

And when you are wounded, you don't always recognize danger—you recognize comfort.

That's how I almost gave my power away.

The church promised healing, but what it slowly introduced was control. Rules disguised as obedience. Fear dressed up as faith. I was told who I could talk to, where I could go, what I could wear, and how I should think. I was so hungry for direction that I mistook domination for discipleship.

I almost lost myself again—this time in the name of God.

My children watched me change. I watched myself shrink. I became afraid to trust my own thoughts. Afraid to question. Afraid to leave. I had already escaped one kind of abuse in my life—I never imagined I would step into another one wearing a different uniform.

But something inside me started to stir.

Not loudly.
Not suddenly.
Slowly.

It began with small doubts. Quiet questions. Moments when what I was being told didn't match what I felt in my spirit. I started realizing that faith shouldn't feel like fear. That God shouldn't feel like intimidation. That healing shouldn't feel like punishment.

I almost stayed silent.

But I didn't.

Leaving wasn't dramatic. It wasn't bold. It was terrifying. Because when you leave something that once felt like your lifeline, you don't just walk away—you fall back into uncertainty. And I had lived in uncertainty my whole life.

But this time, I chose it.

I chose to trust myself for the first time in a long time. I chose to believe that my voice mattered. That my instincts weren't broken. That I didn't need someone else to tell me who I was allowed to become.

That decision didn't fix my life overnight.
It didn't erase my past.
It didn't magically bring success.

But it gave me something I hadn't had in years.

Agency.

I began to see myself differently—not as a victim of circumstance, but as a woman who had survived circumstances that should have destroyed her. I stopped asking,

*Why did this happen to me?* and started asking, *What can I become because of it?*

For the first time, the future didn't feel completely closed.

It still felt far away.
It still felt fragile.
But it felt possible.

I wasn't healed yet.
I wasn't whole yet.
I wasn't confident yet.

But I was no longer lost.

And for someone who had spent her life almost disappearing, that was everything.

# BACK TO SCHOOL

*Almost*

The idea of going back to school didn't come to me like a dream. It came like a dare—one of those quiet challenges life throws at you when you're tired of settling but scared of failing. I didn't wake up one morning believing I could become a doctor. I woke up knowing I couldn't keep living the same life and calling it survival.

For years, education felt like a door I had already closed. I was a high school dropout. A young mother. A woman who had spent more time trying to survive than trying to plan. School belonged to other people—people who had stability, time, and support. People who didn't have to choose between studying and feeding their kids.

I almost told myself it was too late.

Almost believed I had missed my window.
Almost accepted that some dreams are only meant for certain people.

Almost stayed where I was because it felt safer than trying and failing.

But the question wouldn't leave me alone.

*Is this really the life you want your children to see?*

Not the struggle—we had survived that.
But the ceiling.

The limit I had placed on my own future.

So I did something that scared me more than any relationship, more than any job, more than any hard night I had ever endured.

I enrolled.

Walking onto a campus for the first time as an adult felt like stepping into someone else's life. I didn't belong there—or at least that's what my fear kept telling me. I was older than most of the students. I carried a past heavier than my backpack. I sat in classrooms wondering if anyone could see right through me—see the teenage mom, the homeless girl, the woman who had once danced just to survive.

I almost quit in the first semester.

The work was hard. The schedule was harder. Balancing children, bills, and books felt impossible. There were nights

I studied with one eye open, exhaustion pulling me toward sleep while determination kept me upright. I cried more than once over assignments I didn't understand and deadlines I thought I couldn't meet.

But something strange started happening.

I wasn't failing.

Not because I was brilliant.
Not because it was easy.
But because I kept showing up.

Class after class.
Test after test.
Day after day.

And slowly, quietly, something shifted.

I stopped seeing myself as the woman who had messed up her life.
I started seeing myself as the woman who was rebuilding it.

The dream of becoming a doctor didn't arrive with confidence. It arrived with disbelief. I said it out loud once—just to see how it sounded—and immediately laughed at myself. *A doctor?* I barely felt like I belonged in college. But the thought wouldn't leave me. It followed me through lectures. Through late-night study sessions. Through moments when I watched my children sleep and wondered what kind of future I could give them.

I almost kept that dream a secret.

I was afraid people would laugh.
Afraid they would remind me of everything I wasn't.
Afraid they would list all the reasons I couldn't.

But deep down, I knew something.

Every life I had lived up to that point had been preparing me for something bigger. I just didn't know what that something was yet.

I wasn't confident.
I wasn't certain.
I wasn't fearless.

I was just tired of giving up on myself.

And that was enough to take the first step.

# THE MCAT

*Almost*

The closer I got to the dream, the heavier it felt.

Saying I wanted to become a doctor was one thing. Trying to become one was something else entirely. The path was nothing like I imagined. It wasn't inspiring posters and proud speeches—it was rejection, silence, and doors that didn't open, no matter how hard I knocked.

I didn't know the rules. I didn't have mentors. I didn't have connections. I didn't grow up around people who became doctors. I was learning everything late—and learning it alone.

I almost let that stop me.

When I started preparing for the MCAT, the pressure became real in a way that made my chest feel tight every day. This wasn't just another test. This was the gate to a life I wasn't sure I was allowed to want. I studied when I could—at kitchen tables, in libraries, at coffee shops—trying to memorize a future I still couldn't fully see myself living in.

I reached out to doctors, asking if I could shadow them. Most never responded. Some said no. Each unanswered message felt like confirmation of the fear I already carried—*You don't belong here.*

I almost believed them.

There were nights I sat staring at books I barely understood, wondering who I thought I was. I had kids depending on me. Bills piling up. A past that already made everything harder. Why was I chasing something so far away?

Then life did what it always does when you're trying to change—it tested you.

Just months before my MCAT, everything started to unravel again. My oldest son—my rock, my helper, my heartbeat—ended up in trouble. I got the call and felt the ground disappear beneath me. While I was trying to build a future, I was also watching my child fight his own battles. I wanted to quit everything and run to him. I wanted to give up my dream because motherhood felt heavier than ambition.

I almost did.

And then, as if life needed to remind me how fragile everything is, tragedy showed up in the smallest, cruelest way. One morning, walking my daughter to the bus stop, I watched our dog get hit by a car right in front of me. I stood frozen while the world kept moving. It felt like a sign I didn't want to read—that nothing stays safe, that nothing is guaranteed.

I carried that image with me into every study session after that. Every page I turned felt heavier. Every formula felt harder to remember. Grief, fear, exhaustion—they all sat beside me while I tried to prepare for the most important test of my life.

I didn't feel strong.
I didn't feel capable.
I didn't feel ready.

I felt almost done.

But something inside me refused to stop—not because I believed I would succeed, but because I didn't know how to live with myself if I didn't try. I took that test not with confidence, but with courage that barely showed up on time.

And even then, the road didn't open.

There were more setbacks. More moments when the dream felt farther away instead of closer. I applied to programs that said no. I waited for answers that never came. I questioned everything—my intelligence, my timing, my worth.

I almost walked away from medicine entirely.

I told myself maybe this dream wasn't for me. Maybe it was something I was allowed to admire from a distance. Maybe surviving was all I was meant to do.

But late one night, sitting alone in the quiet after my kids went to sleep, I realized something that stopped me cold.

I had already lived through everything that should have broken me.
Abuse.
Homelessness.
Poverty.
Fear.
Loss.

And I was still here.

If I could survive that, I could survive rejection.
If I could survive that, I could survive disappointment.
If I could survive that, I could survive trying again.

So I didn't quit.

Not boldly.
Not confidently.
But stubbornly.

I stayed in the fight—not because I knew I would win, but because I refused to let *almost* become the ending of my story.

# MASTERS PROGRAM

*Almost*

By the time I heard the word *accepted*, I had already trained myself not to celebrate too soon. Life had taught me that good news often comes with a shadow. Still, when the door finally opened—when I was accepted into a biomedical master's program—I sat in silence for a long time, just staring at the message.

Not because I didn't care.
Because I almost didn't believe it.

This wasn't medical school. Not yet. But it was closer than I had ever been. For someone who once thought education was no longer an option, this felt like stepping onto a bridge I never imagined I'd cross.

And still, I was afraid.

Walking into that program felt like walking into a room full of people who already belonged. They spoke the language. They knew the process. They understood the system. I was still translating everything in my head—still learning how to stand in places I once believed were off-limits.

I almost convinced myself I was an imposter.

The classes were harder than anything I had done before. The pace was relentless. The pressure never let up. I watched other students struggle and thought, *If this is hard for them, how am I supposed to survive this?*

There were days I sat in lectures barely breathing, afraid that one mistake would expose me—that one bad test would send me right back to the life I was trying so desperately to outgrow.

And then life tested me again.

In the middle of my program, I got another call—the kind of call that makes your heart fall into your stomach. My oldest son was in trouble again. Jail. Probation violations. More pain layered on top of old wounds. I sat in class that day pretending to listen while my mind raced through every fear I had ever carried as a mother.

I was trying to become something new.
He was fighting not to become what life was pulling him toward.

And I felt torn in half.

I wanted to quit school and go save him. I wanted to abandon my dream because motherhood felt heavier than ambition in that moment. I felt selfish for wanting more when my child needed me so desperately.

I almost walked away.

But something in me understood that this time, quitting wouldn't save either of us. I couldn't fix his life by destroying my own. I couldn't teach him resilience if I modeled surrender.

So I stayed.

I went to class with swollen eyes.
I studied with a broken heart.
I kept moving even when everything inside me wanted to stop.

The program didn't get easier. If anything, it got harder. But slowly—almost without realizing it—I got stronger. Not louder. Not bolder. Just steadier.

I stopped asking if I belonged.
I started asking how far I could go.

Then came another shift.

For the first time in my life, I wasn't just chasing a dream—I was preparing for a calling. The idea of becoming a doctor stopped feeling like a fantasy and started feeling like a responsibility. I didn't want the title. I wanted the ability to help people who felt unseen the way I once had.

Women like me.
Children like mine.
Families who didn't have answers but still had hope.

I realized something quietly, sitting alone one night after my kids had gone to bed.

I wasn't trying to prove I was smart anymore.
I was trying to prove that broken beginnings don't have to write the ending.

And for the first time, I let myself believe that maybe—just maybe—I wasn't chasing something impossible.

Maybe I was becoming something inevitable.

Not because life had been easy.
Not because the path was clear.

But because I had already survived everything that was supposed to stop me.

I wasn't unstoppable.
I wasn't fearless.
I wasn't sure of anything.

I was just a woman who had been almost defeated too many times to quit now.

# MEDICAL SCHOOL

*Almost*

By the time I started applying to medical school, I had learned not to expect smooth roads. I had lived long enough to know that every step forward usually came with a test. Still, nothing prepared me for the waiting.

Waiting is its own kind of suffering.

I sent out applications with hands that shook—not from excitement, but from fear. Fear that my past would outweigh my future. Fear that the teenage mother, the dropout, the woman who once survived by any means necessary, would be louder than the woman I was becoming.

Every time I clicked *submit*, I felt exposed. Like I was handing over my whole life and asking strangers to decide if I was worthy of a second chance.

And then came the silence.

Days passed. Weeks passed. Months passed. Each time my phone buzzed, my heart jumped—only to fall again when it wasn't what I hoped for. I watched other people celebrate acceptances while I practiced patience that didn't come naturally to me.

I almost stopped checking my email.

Not because I didn't care—but because caring hurt.

There were nights I lay awake wondering if I had pushed too far this time. If I had dared to want something that wasn't meant for me. I replayed every mistake I had ever made, every bad choice, every wrong turn, convinced that somewhere in my past was the reason my future was being delayed.

I almost convinced myself that delay meant denial.

And then one day, quietly, without ceremony, the moment came.

An email.
A subject line.
A heartbeat I could hear in my ears.

I opened it slowly—not because I wanted to build suspense, but because I was afraid of being broken if it said no.

It didn't.

I read the words once.
Then again.
Then again.

I was being offered a seat.

Not in a dream.
Not in a fantasy.
In real life.

I didn't scream.
I didn't jump.
I didn't call everyone I knew.

I sat down and cried.

Not the kind of tears that come from happiness alone—but the kind that come from release. From finally letting go of years of doubt, years of shame, years of believing I would always be the exception to the good ending.

In that moment, I thought about the girl I used to be—the scared teenager who ran from home, the young mother who lived in shelters, the woman who almost lost herself trying to survive.

She had no idea this was waiting for her.

Starting medical school didn't feel like arriving. It felt like standing at the edge of something terrifying and beautiful all at once. I walked onto campus on the first day feeling like every version of myself had come with me—the broken ones, the brave ones, the lost ones, the hopeful ones.

I carried them all.

The workload was overwhelming. The responsibility felt heavy. Some days, I wondered if I had made a mistake stepping into something so demanding when my life was already full. I was still a mother. Still paying bills. Still navigating problems that didn't pause just because I was chasing a dream.

There were mornings I wanted to stay in bed.
There were nights I cried from exhaustion.
There were moments I questioned whether I was strong enough to finish what I had started.

I almost quit more than once.

But something had changed in me.

Not confidence.
Not certainty.
Commitment.

I had come too far to let *almost* be the ending.

Not after everything I survived.
Not after everything I endured.
Not after everything I became just to stand here.

And for the first time in my life, I wasn't just surviving anymore.

I was stepping into a future I once believed belonged to someone else.

# IMPOSTER SYNDROME

*Almost*

Medical school did not feel like a victory. It felt like war.

Not the kind with noise and headlines—but the quiet kind that happens in your mind at two in the morning when you're staring at notes you don't understand, wondering if you made a mistake believing you could do this. Every lecture felt like drinking from a fire hose. Every exam felt like judgment. And every day carried the weight of knowing that if I failed, I wouldn't just disappoint myself—I would confirm every fear I had ever had about my limits.

I almost let that pressure crush me.

Some of my classmates seemed built for this world. They spoke confidently. They asked the right questions. They looked like they belonged. I sat among them, wondering how a girl who once lived in shelters ended up in the same room as future doctors.

Imposter syndrome didn't whisper—it shouted.

There were nights I cried in my car before driving home because I didn't want my children to see how scared I was. I didn't want them to know that their mother—the woman who kept telling them anything was possible—was afraid she might be lying.

But every morning, I showed up anyway.

Not because I felt ready.
Not because I felt brave.
But because I had learned something over the years—fear doesn't disappear when you wait for it to. It fades when you walk through it.

The pressure didn't stop outside the classroom. Life still demanded its share. Bills. Sick kids. Court dates. School meetings. Broken appliances. Everyday problems that don't pause just because you're chasing a dream. Some days, I studied with one child asleep on my shoulder and another waiting for dinner on the stove.

I almost burned out.

There were moments when quitting felt logical. When going back to a simpler life felt tempting. When the idea of being "just okay" seemed easier than fighting for "extraordinary."

But then I would remember who I used to be.

The girl who ran from home.
The young mother who lived in shelters.
The woman who survived abuse and poverty.

She didn't survive all of that for me to quit now.

Slowly, something changed.

Not overnight.
Not dramatically.
But steadily.

I stopped measuring myself against everyone else. I stopped trying to prove I deserved to be there. I focused on the only thing I could control—my effort. One lecture at a time. One test at a time. One exhausted day at a time.

And then came the moments that made it all worth it.

The first patient interaction.
The first time someone thanked me for listening.

The first time I realized I wasn't just learning medicine—I was becoming a healer.

I thought back to every version of myself that had felt invisible, voiceless, powerless. I understood then why this path had called me so relentlessly. I wasn't here by accident. I wasn't here by luck. I was here because life had prepared me to care for people in a way textbooks never could.

Still, I never felt safe celebrating.

Every milestone felt fragile—like something that could be taken away at any moment. I had lived too long waiting for the other shoe to drop. I had survived too many good moments that were followed by hard ones.

So I kept my head down.
I kept working.
I kept going.

And then, one quiet day, it happened.

I stood in a room wearing a white coat.

Not as a dream.
Not as a fantasy.
But as reality.

I didn't feel proud at first. I felt stunned.

Because I knew exactly how close I had come to never being there at all.

I wasn't unstoppable.
I wasn't fearless.
I wasn't special.

I was almost broken too many times to count.

And somehow, still standing.

# DOCTOR

*Almost*

The first day I walked into work as a doctor didn't feel like the movies.

There was no slow-motion moment.
No swelling music.
No crowd applauding.

There was just me—standing in a hallway that smelled like disinfectant and coffee, wearing a white coat that still didn't feel real, holding a badge with my name on it and a title I never thought would belong to me.

Doctor.

I stared at that badge longer than I should have. Not because I was proud—but because I was stunned. Because I knew exactly how many versions of my life never made it to this hallway. How many endings could have stopped me long before this beginning.

I thought about the girl who ran from home.
The teenager who lived in shelters.
The young mother who counted dollars at grocery stores.
The woman who stayed in places she should have fled.
The student who almost quit more times than she admitted.

They were all still with me.

I carried them into every patient room. Into every chart I opened. Into every conversation I had with someone who was scared, hurting, or uncertain about their future. I understood fear in a way textbooks never taught. I understood survival in a way no lecture could explain.

And for the first time in my life, I realized something quietly powerful.

Nothing I had lived through was wasted.

Every painful chapter had trained me to see people—not just symptoms. To listen—not just hear. To care—not just cure. I didn't become a doctor despite my past. I became one because of it.

Still, I didn't feel finished.

Success didn't erase the past. It didn't heal every wound. It didn't give me back the years I lost trying to survive. But it gave me something I never thought I'd have.

Perspective.

I stopped asking why my life had been so hard and started understanding what it had shaped me to become. Strength wasn't loud. It wasn't flashy. It was quiet. Consistent. Relentless.

It was getting up one more time than you fell.
It was choosing yourself when no one else did.
It was refusing to let *almost* become the end of your story.

Sometimes I look back and think about how close I came.

Almost gave up.
Almost stayed broken.
Almost believed the lies.
Almost disappeared.

But I didn't.

And if you're reading this, wondering whether your life can still change—if you feel like you've waited too long, messed up too much, or missed your moment—I need you to hear this from someone who lived it:

Almost is not the end.
Almost is the edge.
Almost is the place where everything can still turn around.

I wasn't unstoppable.

I was almost lost.

And somehow—still here.

# PART II – BECOMING

*Almost*

For a long time, I thought becoming a doctor would feel like arriving.

Like everything that hurt before would finally make sense.
Like the weight I carried for years would lift.
Like, I would finally be free.

But becoming didn't feel like freedom.

It felt like starting over — again.

Because when you spend your whole life surviving, you don't automatically know how to live once the danger is gone. You know how to fight. You know how to endure. You know how to push. But peace feels unfamiliar. Stability feels suspicious. Happiness feels like something you're waiting to lose.

I didn't step into my new life with confidence.
I stepped into it carefully — like someone walking on thin ice.

I had a title now. A career that people respected. A story people admired. But inside, I was still the girl who learned to sleep lightly because safety never lasted long. Still, the woman who waited for the next bad thing to happen because it always used to.

Success didn't erase that.

Some nights I lie awake thinking, *What if this all disappears?*
What if I lose this too?
What if I don't deserve this?

I had spent years proving I could survive hardship.
Now I had to learn how to survive **peace**.

And that was harder than anything I expected.

People looked at me differently now. They saw strength. They saw resilience. They saw inspiration. They didn't see the exhaustion that still lived in my bones. They didn't see how heavy it felt to carry a past that didn't match my present.

I had changed — but the world hadn't changed with me.

Some people clung to the old version of me.
Some resented the new one.
Some couldn't understand how a woman with my story now stood where I stood.

And sometimes... neither could I.

There were days I walked into work and felt like I was playing a role I hadn't fully grown into yet. Not because I wasn't capable — but because I had never seen anyone like me in spaces like this before. I had no mirror for this version of myself.

So I became my own.

I learned that becoming isn't loud.
It isn't flashy.
It isn't instant.

Becoming is quiet work.

It's choosing healing when you're used to pain.
It's choosing rest when you're used to running.
It's choosing joy when you're used to bracing for loss.

I had spent years almost breaking.

Now I had to learn how not to break when life finally gave me something good.

And slowly — almost without realizing it — I started to live in a way I never had before.

Not just surviving.
Not just enduring.
But breathing.

For the first time in my life, I wasn't standing on the edge of collapse.
I was standing on the edge of becoming someone I had never imagined I could be.

And even then... I still whispered the same word to myself when things felt fragile.

Almost.

Not as fear anymore.
But as faith.

Almost lost — but found.
Almost broken — but healed.
Almost gone — but still here.

And this time... I wasn't just surviving my life.

I was finally living it.

We keep going.

# SURVIVAL MODE

*Almost*

When people hear my story now, they think the hardest part was becoming a doctor.
They think the struggle ended the day I put on that white coat.

They're wrong.

The hardest part came after.

Because once the noise of survival quiets down, you finally hear everything you've been carrying. All the fear you pushed aside. All the pain you buried under busyness. All the wounds you never had time to tend because you were too busy staying alive.

I had built a life on endurance.
I didn't know how to build one on peace.

For years, my body had been trained for stress. My mind had learned to live on alert. Even when life finally slowed down, I didn't. I still flinched at sudden changes. Still braced myself for bad news. Still waited for something to go wrong.

Sometimes, in the middle of good moments, I felt uneasy.
Not because I wasn't grateful.
But because happiness felt unfamiliar.

I had lived too long in chaos to trust calm.

There were days I sat alone in my car after work, staring at the steering wheel, asking myself questions I never thought I'd have time to ask.

Who am I when I'm not fighting anymore?
Who am I when I'm not proving myself?
Who am I when I don't have to be strong every second of the day?

I didn't have answers yet.

All I knew was that I didn't want to live the rest of my life still shaped by everything that almost destroyed me.

So I started doing the work I had avoided for years.

Not schoolwork.
Not career work.
Soul work.

I faced memories I had locked away.
I forgave people I once swore I never would.
I learned how to forgive myself — for staying too long, for running too far, for believing lies I had been taught to believe about my worth.

That was the hardest healing of all.

There were moments when I felt like I was breaking all over again — not because life was hurting me, but because I was finally letting myself feel what I had been numb to for so long.

Healing isn't pretty.
It isn't neat.
It doesn't follow a schedule.

Some days I felt strong.
Some days I felt small.
Some days I felt proud.
Some days I felt ashamed.

But for the first time, I stayed present for all of it.

I stopped running from discomfort.
I stopped numbing pain with busyness.
I stopped pretending I was fine when I wasn't.

And slowly, I learned something that changed everything.

Strength isn't only built in hardship.
Strength is built in honesty.

I didn't need to be the woman who survived everything anymore.
I needed to become the woman who could finally rest.

Not collapse.
Rest.

There is a difference.

Collapsing comes from exhaustion.
Rest comes from safety.

And I was finally learning what safety felt like.

Not perfect safety.
Not guaranteed safety.
But enough to breathe without fear every second of the day.

I started building a life that wasn't just impressive — but peaceful.
A life that didn't just look good from the outside — but felt good on the inside.

And that's when I realized something quietly powerful.

The girl who almost gave up...
The woman who almost stayed broken...
The mother who almost lost herself...

She didn't survive all of that just to be successful.

She survived it to be whole.

And that — more than any title, any degree, any achievement — is what becoming really means.

# LETTING GO

*Almost*

One of the strangest parts of becoming someone new is realizing how many people still expect you to be who you used to be.

I didn't change overnight. But I did change deeply. And not everyone was ready for that.

Some people celebrated my growth.
Some people questioned it.
Some people resented it.

And some people tried to pull me back into the version of myself that made them comfortable.

I had spent most of my life shrinking to fit into other people's expectations—being quiet when I wanted to speak, being agreeable when I wanted to stand firm, being grateful when I wanted to demand more. Survival teaches you how to adapt. It doesn't teach you how to lead.

Becoming required something different.

It required boundaries.

That was new for me.

For years, I had believed that love meant endurance. That loyalty meant staying. That strength meant tolerating pain. I had mistaken patience for purpose and sacrifice for destiny.

But as I healed, I began to see clearly for the first time.

Love does not require suffering.
Loyalty does not demand silence.
Strength does not mean self-erasure.

Those realizations changed everything.

I started saying no without apologizing.
I started choosing myself without guilt.
I started walking away from conversations that drained me instead of trying to fix them.

And that felt dangerous at first.

Because when you've lived your whole life in reaction mode, choosing yourself feels selfish. When you've survived by pleasing others, protecting your peace feels rebellious.

I almost went back to my old ways.

Almost told myself I was being too much.
Almost convinced myself I was asking for too much.
Almost shrank again to make everyone else comfortable.

But I didn't.

For the first time in my life, I trusted the woman I was becoming more than the woman I used to be.

That changed my relationships.

Some people grew closer.
Some people drifted away.
Some chapters closed quietly.

And I learned something that took me years to understand:

Not every loss is a loss.

Some endings are protection.

Some goodbyes are answers to prayers you were too afraid to pray out loud.

Letting go didn't feel empowering at first. It felt lonely. It felt like standing in a new version of my life without a map. But slowly, the loneliness turned into peace. And the peace turned into clarity.

I began to see myself not as a woman who had survived a hard life—but as a woman who was finally choosing a good one.

Not perfect.
Not painless.
But intentional.

I started dreaming differently.

Not about escaping anymore.
Not about proving anything.
But about building something that would last.

A life my children could feel safe inside.
A future that didn't require constant fighting.
A legacy built on healing instead of hurt.

I wasn't running anymore.

I wasn't hiding anymore.

I wasn't waiting for disaster anymore.

I was standing in the middle of my life and realizing something that made me pause.

I didn't almost make it.

I did.

And now... I finally had the courage to live like it.

# PEACE

## *Almost*

For the first time in my life, I wasn't running toward something anymore.

I was standing still long enough to build.

That was new for me.

For years, my life had been about escape—escaping fear, escaping poverty, escaping pain, escaping the version of myself I didn't want to be. But when the danger finally faded, I realized something quietly unsettling.

I didn't know how to live without running.

So I had to learn.

I started paying attention to the moments I used to rush past—the mornings when my children laughed over breakfast, the evenings when the house finally felt calm, the silence that no longer felt lonely but peaceful. I realized I had spent so much of my life bracing for impact that I never fully felt the joy when it finally arrived.

I had almost missed that too.

Motherhood felt different now. Not heavy in the same way. Not desperate. Not driven by fear. I wasn't parenting from survival anymore—I was parenting from stability. From presence. From the deep understanding of what my children had seen me overcome.

They didn't just watch me survive.

They watched me become.

And that changed how I saw myself as their mother. I wasn't just raising children anymore—I was raising witnesses. Witnesses to resilience. Witnesses to healing. Witnesses to the truth that your beginnings don't get the final word.

Sometimes I would catch my reflection in the mirror and barely recognize the woman looking back at me. Not because she was unrecognizable—but because she was finally at peace.

I had spent most of my life almost breaking.

Now I was learning how not to.

I began speaking to women who reminded me of myself—the ones still stuck in the middle, still fighting to breathe, still believing they were too far gone. I didn't speak to them as a success story. I spoke to them as a survivor who understood exactly how close they were to disappearing.

I told them the truth.

That strength isn't glamorous.
That healing isn't fast.
That transformation doesn't announce itself.

It happens quietly. In choices no one applauds. In courage no one sees.

I reminded them that almost doesn't mean failure.

Almost means you were close to giving up — and you didn't.
Almost means you were near the edge — and you stepped back.
Almost means the story could have ended — and it didn't.

That word changed for me over time.

Almost used to feel like regret.
Now it feels like grace.

Grace that carried me through places I wasn't supposed to survive.

Grace that held me when I had nothing left to give.
Grace that waited for me to believe in myself again.

And when I think about everything I lived through, everything I almost lost, everything I almost became — I understand something now that I couldn't see then.

My life was never about being unstoppable.

It was about being *still here.*

Still standing.
Still choosing.
Still healing.
Still loving.
Still becoming.

And if you're reading this while standing in your own *almost* — tired, scared, uncertain — I want you to know something I learned the hard way.

You don't have to have it all together.
You don't have to feel brave.
You don't have to know the ending.

You just have to stay.

Stay when it hurts.
Stay when you doubt yourself.
Stay when the past whispers that you're done.

Because sometimes the greatest victory isn't making it big.

Sometimes the greatest victory is simply...

Not leaving your own life.

# PART III – STILL HERE

*Almost*

There was a time when I thought surviving meant winning.

I thought if I could just get out...
If I could just make it through...
If I could just become something different...

then everything would finally feel whole.

But survival is only the beginning.

Living is the work that comes after.

For a long time, I carried my story like armor. I told it to prove I was strong. I told it to show I had overcome. I told it so no one would ever mistake me for weak again.

But now, I tell it for a different reason.

I tell it because I almost didn't make it.

Not in the dramatic way people imagine.
Not in one moment.
In a thousand quiet ones.

I almost stayed in places that were killing me.
I almost believed lies that would have kept me small.
I almost accepted a life I was never meant to live.
I almost stopped dreaming because dreaming hurt too much.

Almost is not failure.

Almost is the space between who you were and who you could still become.

Most people never talk about that space.
They either talk about the fall...
or the victory.

But not the middle.

The middle is where I lived most of my life.
And maybe you do too.

The middle is messy.
The middle is exhausting.
The middle is lonely.
The middle is where you question everything you thought you knew about yourself.

And yet — the middle is where transformation actually happens.

Not when everything is fixed.
Not when everything makes sense.
But when you are tired, uncertain, and still choosing to wake up one more day.

I used to think strength looked like never breaking.

Now I know strength looks like breaking — and staying.

Staying in your life when it hurts.
Staying in your healing when it's uncomfortable.
Staying in your growth when it scares you.

Staying when leaving would be easier.

There are still days when I look back and feel the weight of what I lost — time, innocence, peace I didn't get to have when others did. There are still moments when I wonder who I would be if life had been kinder to me earlier.

But I don't live there anymore.

I live here.

In the woman I became.
In the mother I learned to be.

In the peace I fought for.
In the future I almost never believed I deserved.

And when I think about everything I survived — everything I almost became — I no longer see a story about being unstoppable.

I see a story about being **still here**.

Still loving.
Still trying.
Still growing.
Still choosing life.

If you are reading this while standing in your own almost — almost giving up, almost settling, almost believing the worst about yourself — I need you to hear this in a way I wish someone had told me years ago.

You don't have to be fearless.
You don't have to be perfect.
You don't have to be unstoppable.

You just have to stay.

Stay when the road is unclear.
Stay when your past tries to pull you back.
Stay when your future feels too far away to reach.

Because sometimes the bravest thing you will ever do...

is not disappear.

# THE REFLECTION GUIDE

You've just finished reading a story about survival, becoming, and staying.

Not a perfect story.
Not a polished one.
A real one.

Now this part of the book invites you to do something different.

Not just read.
But **reflect**.

Because stories don't change lives on their own.
**Understanding does.**
**Action does.**
**Choice does.**

This section exists for one reason:

To help you turn what you felt while reading...
into what you **do** after reading.

The chapters that follow are not here to fix you.
They are here to **walk with you**.

Each reflection section is built around three simple movements:

1. **Insight** — understanding what the chapter really revealed
2. **Lessons** — the truths that rise from the story
3. **To-Do Lists** — small, real steps toward change

No pressure.
No perfection required.
Just honesty.

You don't have to complete every exercise.
You don't have to move fast.
You don't even have to feel ready.

You only have to be willing to look at your life with the same courage you used to read this story.

Because if *Almost* has shown you anything, it's this:

Transformation doesn't begin when everything is clear.
It begins when you decide not to stay where you are.

This Reflection Guide is not about becoming someone else.
It's about becoming **more of who you already are**.

The you who survived.
The you who stayed.
The you who almost gave up—but didn't.

Take what serves you.
Leave what doesn't.
Move at your own pace.

There is no right way to heal.
There is only your way forward.

And if you are still here...
that means your story is still being written.

Let's keep building it—together.

# HIGH SCHOOL

## Reflection

This chapter isn't just about a hard childhood.
It's about how **survival trains us**.

When you grow up in instability, your nervous system learns to stay on guard. You learn to read rooms before you read books. You learn to sense danger before you understand love. You grow up fast—not because you want to, but because you have to.

In *Broken Childhood*, you see how pain doesn't always arrive loudly. Sometimes it comes quietly—through absence, through confusion, through wanting to be loved more than wanting to be safe. And when that happens early enough, you don't recognize damage as damage. You recognize it as normal.

This chapter shows how:

- Abuse gets mistaken for affection
- Fear gets mistaken for loyalty
- Survival gets mistaken for strength

And yet... it also shows something else.

Even in the middle of confusion, something inside you knew this wasn't the life you were meant to live. You didn't have language for it yet. You didn't have a plan. But you had **instinct**—the quiet voice that kept telling you, *This isn't the end of your story.*

That voice is what saved you long before success ever did.

## The Lessons

1. **What feels normal is not always healthy.**
   Just because pain is familiar doesn't mean it's right.
2. **Survival is not the same as safety.**
   You can survive something that is still destroying you.
3. **Abuse teaches the wrong definition of love.**
   Real love does not hurt, threaten, or control.
4. **You can be strong and still need help.**
   Independence learned through trauma is often loneliness in disguise.

5. **Your beginnings influence you—but they do not own you.**
   Where you started explains you. It does not limit you.
6. **Instinct is the first form of wisdom.**
   Long before you had clarity, you had a feeling that there was more for you. That mattered.

## The To-Do List

If this chapter felt personal to you, start here.

### 1. Name what you normalized

Write down three things from your past that once felt "normal" but you now realize were harmful or unhealthy.

Examples:

- Staying in situations that scared you
- Accepting disrespect
- Thinking love meant pain

Awareness is the first step out of patterns.

## 2. Redefine love

Complete this sentence in writing:

> "Love is not ________. Love is ________."

Do this for yourself—not for anyone else.

## 3. Identify your survival habits

List three habits you developed just to get through life that may no longer serve you.

Examples:

- Shutting down emotionally
- Overworking
- People-pleasing
- Staying silent to keep peace

Circle one you are ready to outgrow.

## 4. Choose one boundary

Ask yourself:

> "What is one boundary I wish I had learned sooner?"

Write it down. Practice saying it out loud.

### 5. Speak one truth

Find one safe person—or a journal—and finally say one thing you've always carried quietly.

Healing begins where silence ends.

## Closing Reflection

You were not weak for what you endured.
You were not foolish for what you didn't understand yet.
You were not broken beyond repair.

You were a child learning how to survive in a world that should have protected you better.

And the fact that you are still here means something powerful:

You were always more than your circumstances.
You were always more than your past.
You were always more than the life you almost accepted.

This chapter isn't about what hurt you.

It's about what **couldn't stop you** — even when you didn't know how to stop it yet.

# PREGNANCY

## Reflection

This chapter shows what happens when trauma doesn't just shape how you feel — it shapes how you **choose**. When you grow up learning to survive, you don't always choose what's best for you. You choose what feels familiar. You choose what feels fast. You choose what feels like relief.

Not because you're reckless.
But because you're tired.

This chapter reveals how desperation doesn't always look like despair. Sometimes it looks like opportunity. Sometimes it looks like freedom. Sometimes it looks like money, attention, or escape. And when you've lived in lack long enough, anything that promises ease feels like salvation.

You weren't chasing danger.
You were chasing **rest**.

This chapter also shows something many people never talk about:

Survival can turn into a trap.

When you learn how to make it through anything, you start believing you have to. You stop asking if a life is healthy and start asking only if it's **possible**. And that's how people stay in places that slowly erase them.

But this chapter also shows the turning point.

The moment when you finally saw yourself clearly.
Not as strong.
Not as empowered.
But as worthy of more.

That moment wasn't loud.
It was honest.

And honesty is where real change begins.

## The Lessons

1. **Desperation doesn't make you weak — it makes you vulnerable.**
   Vulnerability needs protection, not judgment.

2. **Fast relief is rarely real freedom.**
   Anything that saves you today but costs you tomorrow is not rescue — it's delay.
3. **Survival skills can become self-sabotage.**
   What once kept you alive can later keep you stuck.
4. **Attention is not affection.**
   Being seen is not the same as being valued.
5. **You don't leave unhealthy places because you feel strong.**
   You leave when you finally feel tired enough to choose yourself.
6. **Freedom begins with clarity, not courage.**
   You don't need boldness first — you need truth.

## The To-Do List

If this chapter spoke to you, this is your starting place.

### 1. Identify your escape patterns

Answer honestly:

> "When life feels overwhelming, I usually escape by ___________."

Examples:

- Working nonstop

- Spending money you don't have
- Entering unhealthy relationships
- Numbing with substances or distractions

Write it down without judging yourself.

## 2. Separate relief from healing

| What brings relief | What brings healing |
|---|---|
| Relief feels good now. | Healing feels better later. |

Notice the difference.

## 3. Reclaim your worth

Finish this sentence in writing:

> "I am worth more than the life I have been settling for."

Read it every day for a week.

## 4. Choose one honest exit

Ask yourself:

> "What is one situation in my life that I've stayed in because it was familiar — not because it was healthy?"

You don't have to leave today.
But you do need to **tell yourself the truth** about it.

### 5. Make one clean choice

Choose one small action this week that supports the life you want — not just the life you've been surviving.

Examples:

- Applying for something better
- Saying no to something draining
- Asking for help
- Setting one boundary

Growth doesn't start big.
It starts **true.**

## Closing Reflection

You were never reckless.
You were exhausted.

You were never weak.
You were surviving without a safety net.

And when survival is all you know, freedom feels foreign.

But the moment you stopped accepting the life that was killing you slowly — even without a plan — you proved something powerful:

You were never trapped.
You were just tired of running.

And tired people who finally choose themselves...
change their lives.

# THE STRIP CLUB

## Reflection

## What This Chapter Really Shows

Part III is about the moment when survival finally turns into **choice**.

This chapter isn't about escape anymore.
It's about awakening.

It shows what happens when you stop asking, *How do I get through this?*
and start asking, *Why am I still living like this?*

That shift is everything.

Most people don't change when life is painful — they change when life becomes **unacceptable**. When you reach the point where survival no longer feels brave, it feels expensive. Expensive to your peace. Expensive to your future. Expensive to your children.

This chapter shows the moment you finally chose **self-respect over familiarity**.

You didn't leave because you were confident.
You left because you were **done**.

Done running.
Done hiding.
Done shrinking.
Done convincing yourself that this was all life would ever be.

That decision didn't come with certainty.
It came with **clarity**.

And clarity is the beginning of freedom.

## The Lessons

1. **You don't change when you feel ready. You change when you feel finished.**
   Finished tolerating. Finished excusing. Finished surviving.

2. **Familiar pain feels safer than unfamiliar peace — until it doesn't.**
   Growth always begins with discomfort.
3. **Choosing yourself feels selfish to people who benefited from your silence.**
   That does not make it wrong.
4. **The hardest boundary is the one you set with your past.**
   But it is also the most powerful.
5. **You don't need confidence to leave — you need clarity.**
   Courage comes after the decision.
6. **Your future starts the moment you stop negotiating with your worth.**

## The To-Do List

If this chapter felt close to home, this is your next step forward.

### 1. Write your "I'm done" list

Finish this sentence three times:

"I am done ___________."

Examples:

- I am done explaining myself.
- I am done accepting less.
- I am done surviving when I could be living.

## 2. Identify what you've outgrown

Answer honestly:

> "What part of my life feels familiar but no longer fits who I am becoming?"

Write it down. That's your clarity.

## 3. Practice choosing yourself

This week, do **one thing** that honors your peace.

Examples:

- Cancel something draining
- Say no without explanation
- Ask for what you need
- Walk away from a situation that hurts

Growth doesn't come from bold moves — it comes from honest ones.

### 4. Rewrite your identity

Complete this sentence:

> "I am no longer the person who __________.
> I am becoming the person who __________."

Read it every morning for seven days.

### 5. Make peace with discomfort

Say this to yourself out loud:

> "This feels uncomfortable because I am growing — not because I am wrong."

Let discomfort become your confirmation, not your warning.

## Closing Reflection

You didn't change your life because it got easier.
You changed your life because **you got clearer**.

Clearer about what you deserved.
Clearer about what you would no longer accept.
Clearer about who you were tired of being.

And that clarity did what strength alone never could.

It freed you.

This chapter is proof that your life didn't turn because you were fearless.
It turned because you were finally honest.

And honesty is the birthplace of every real transformation.

You were never meant to live in survival forever.
You were meant to **outgrow** it.

And you did.

# MARRIAGE

## Reflection

This chapter shows the quiet, confusing space between leaving a hard life and actually building a new one. Most people think the hardest part is escaping what hurts you. But often, the hardest part is learning how to live once the danger is gone.

This chapter of my life reveals a truth many people never say out loud:

Freedom can feel empty at first.

When you've lived your whole life reacting to crisis, peace feels strange. Stability feels boring. Calm feels suspicious. You don't know who you are without chaos pushing you forward.

So instead of celebrating escape, you start questioning it.

*Did I make the right choice?*
*Was I stronger in survival mode?*
*Who am I now that I'm not just fighting anymore?*

This chapter shows the moment when you stop measuring your life by what you escaped...
and start measuring it by what you are building.

Not fast.
Not perfectly.
But intentionally.

And that shift is the beginning of **true change**.

## The Lessons

1. **Leaving survival doesn't mean you immediately feel free.**
   Freedom often starts as confusion before it becomes peace.
2. **Chaos can feel more comfortable than calm.**
   Familiar pain is easier than unfamiliar stability.
3. **Starting over is lonely — but it is also powerful.**
   Growth often begins in quiet spaces where no one is watching.

4. **You don't need a clear future to move forward.**
   You just need a different direction than before.
5. **Rebuilding your life also means rebuilding your identity.**
   You are not who you were when you were just surviving.
6. **Progress isn't loud.**
   Sometimes the biggest change is simply choosing not to go backward.

## The To-Do List

If this chapter felt personal, this is your next step.

### 1. Name what you left behind

Write down one part of your life you escaped that still tries to pull you back emotionally.

Then write this sentence:

> "I left because I deserved more than survival."

Read it out loud.

## 2. Identify your discomfort with peace

Answer honestly:

> "What feels strange or uncomfortable about stability in my life right now?"

Sometimes discomfort isn't a warning — it's a sign you're growing.

## 3. Redefine who you are becoming

Complete this sentence:

> "I am no longer building my life around ___________. I am building my life around ___________."

Examples:

- fear → peace
- reaction → intention
- survival → growth

## 4. Practice choosing progress

This week, choose **one small habit** that supports your future instead of your past.

Examples:

- saving a small amount of money
- showing up on time
- applying for something new
- leaving a draining conversation early

Growth begins with consistency, not perfection.

### 5. Write your new direction

Answer this in your journal:

> "If I could build a life that feels safe and fulfilling, it would look like ___________."

Don't worry about how yet.
Vision comes before strategy.

## Closing Reflection

You didn't escape your old life just to wander.

You escaped so you could **build**.

Build peace where there was panic.
Build direction where there was confusion.
Build hope where there was only endurance.

This chapter is not about the moment you left.

It's about the moment you decided to **move forward** —
even when you didn't yet know where forward would lead.

That decision is the first quiet victory of your new life.

And quiet victories...
are the ones that last.

# THE CHURCH

## Reflection

This chapter shows the transition from simply leaving a hard life to finally **learning from it**.

Many people escape their past physically but never leave it emotionally. They change environments, relationships, even identities — yet the old wounds still make the decisions. Fear still speaks louder than hope. Doubt still feels safer than belief.

This chapter shows the moment you began to realize:

You weren't just running from what hurt you.
You were being called toward who you were becoming.

That shift is subtle, but it is powerful.

It's the moment you stop asking, *Why did this happen to me?*
and start asking, *What can I build because I survived it?*

This chapter reveals that healing doesn't start when life gets easier.
Healing starts when you finally stop avoiding your own story.

## The Lessons

1. **You can leave a place and still live there emotionally.**
   True freedom means healing, not just escaping.
2. **Understanding your past gives you power over it.**
   What you can name, you can change.
3. **Pain doesn't disqualify you — it prepares you.**
   Your struggle trained you in ways comfort never could.
4. **Growth begins when you stop asking who hurt you and start asking who you are becoming.**
5. **You don't need to erase your story to rise above it.**
   You need to learn from it.
6. **Your past is a chapter — not the whole book.**

## The To-Do List

If this chapter stirred something in you, begin here.

### 1. Separate who you were from who you are

Finish this sentence in writing:

> "I am not the person I was when ________."

Read it slowly. Let yourself believe it.

### 2. Name the lesson in the pain

Answer honestly:

> "The hardest season of my life taught me __________."

Turn your pain into purpose by naming what it gave you.

### 3. Reclaim your narrative

Write one paragraph answering this question:

> "If I could tell my story from a place of strength instead of shame, I would say __________."

Your story changes when your voice changes.

### 4. Choose growth over guilt

This week, release **one guilt** you've been carrying from your past.

Write it down. Then write this under it:

> "I forgive myself for surviving the only way I knew how."

### 5. Take one step toward your future

Ask yourself:

> "What is one action I can take this month that my past version of me never believed was possible?"

Do that.

## Closing Reflection

You did not survive your childhood just to spend the rest of your life apologizing for it.

You survived so you could **outgrow** it.

You survived so you could rewrite the ending.
You survived so you could become proof that beginnings don't decide destinies.

This chapter is not about what you went through.

It's about what you are becoming because you did.

And that is the difference between living in your past...
and building from it.

# BACK TO SCHOOL

## Reflection

This chapter shows what happens when life stops being only about you—and becomes about who is watching you. For many people, real change doesn't begin when they decide they deserve better. It begins when they realize someone else is learning from them.

This is the chapter where survival turns into **example**.

You weren't just fighting for your own future anymore.
You were shaping someone else's.

That shift changes everything.

It changes how you make decisions.
It changes what you tolerate.
It changes what you accept as "normal."

This chapter shows how love—real love—forces growth. Not the kind that feels good at first, but the kind that feels heavy because it carries responsibility.

And responsibility is the doorway to maturity.

## The Lessons

1. **You rise differently when someone depends on you.**
   Responsibility can unlock strength you never knew you had.
2. **Breaking cycles starts with awareness.**
   You can't change what you don't first recognize.
3. **Your choices teach even when you are silent.**
   Children learn more from what we live than from what we say.
4. **Love that heals requires courage.**
   It takes bravery to become the person your family needs.
5. **You don't have to be perfect to be powerful.**
   You only have to be present and intentional.
6. **Legacy begins long before success.**
   It starts the moment you choose growth over comfort.

## The To-Do List

If this chapter connected with you, start here.

### 1. Identify who you're influencing

Write down the names of the people who are watching your life—children, siblings, friends, coworkers.

Then answer:

> "What are they learning from the way I live right now?"

### 2. Break one cycle

Ask yourself:

> "What pattern in my family or life do I want to end with me?"

Write it down. That's your mission.

### 3. Redefine responsibility

Finish this sentence:

> "Being responsible now means __________."

Let responsibility become empowerment, not pressure.

### 4. Choose one example to set

This week, intentionally model one value:

- honesty
- consistency
- patience
- courage
- self-respect

Do it on purpose.

### 5. Write your legacy statement

Complete this sentence:

> "When people look at my life, I want them to see ___________."

Keep it simple. Keep it true.

## Closing Reflection

You didn't rise because life finally got easier.
You rose because someone needed you to.

And in becoming what they needed...
you became who you were meant to be.

This chapter is not just about responsibility.

It's about **transformation through love**.

And that kind of transformation lasts longer than any success story ever could.

# THE MCAT

## Reflection

This chapter shows what happens when you start to believe your life can change—after years of disappointment. When you've been let down enough times, hope doesn't feel inspiring anymore. It feels risky. It feels like something you don't want to touch, because if you believe again and fail again, it hurts even more.

So many people stop dreaming not because they don't want more...
but because they're tired of being disappointed.

This chapter reveals the quiet battle between two voices:

The voice that says, *Don't get your hopes up.*
And the voice that says, *But what if this time is different?*

Growth happens when you choose to listen to the second voice—even when it trembles.

## The Lessons

1. **Disappointment trains you to expect less—but you don't have to live that way forever.**
   Your past failures do not get to decide your future expectations.
2. **Hope feels scary when you've been hurt too many times.**
   That fear doesn't mean you're weak—it means you're human.
3. **Believing again is an act of courage.**
   It takes strength to risk your heart on a better future.
4. **You don't need certainty to move forward.**
   You need willingness.
5. **Cynicism feels safe—but it keeps you small.**
   Hope feels risky—but it makes you grow.
6. **The future changes the moment you decide not to give up on it.**

## The To-Do List

If this chapter felt close to home, start here.

### 1. Name what you stopped hoping for

Finish this sentence:

> "I stopped hoping for __________ because __________."

Be honest. There is no shame in fatigue.

### 2. Challenge your fear of disappointment

Ask yourself:

> "What am I more afraid of—failing again or never trying again?"

Write your answer. Sit with it.

### 3. Choose one small hope

Pick **one thing** you will allow yourself to believe in again.
Not everything. Just one.

Examples:

- A healthier relationship
- A better job
- Emotional peace
- A fresh start

## 4. Take one hopeful action

This week, do one thing that supports the life you want—not the life you fear.

Examples:

- Apply
- Reach out
- Start saving
- Say yes to an opportunity
- Say no to a limitation

Hope grows when action follows belief.

## 5. Write your permission slip

Write this sentence and sign it:

> "I give myself permission to believe that my life can still become something beautiful."

Put your name under it.

## Closing Reflection

You were never afraid of dreaming.
You were afraid of being hurt again.

But healing doesn't come from protecting yourself from hope.
It comes from letting yourself believe—slowly, carefully, bravely—that your story isn't finished.

This chapter is not about sudden confidence.
It's about **quiet courage**.

The courage to hope again.
The courage to try again.
The courage to believe that *almost* isn't the end—
it's the place where a new beginning can finally start.

# MASTERS PROGRAM

## Reflection

Not your circumstances yet.
Not your bank account yet.
Not your title yet.

But **you**.

This chapter shows the quiet internal shift that happens when you stop seeing yourself only as someone who survived—and start seeing yourself as someone who can **become**.

For a long time, survival had been your identity.
Strong. Tough. Independent. Unbreakable.

But underneath that strength was exhaustion.

This chapter reveals the moment you realized that being strong all the time was no longer a badge of honor—it was a burden. You didn't need to prove you could survive anymore. You needed to learn how to **receive** support, growth, and opportunity.

That shift is the beginning of transformation.

Not when life changes.
But when your **self-image** does.

## The Lessons

1. **You outgrow survival before you outgrow struggle.**
   Growth starts on the inside long before it shows on the outside.
2. **Strength without healing becomes exhaustion.**
   You deserve rest—not just resilience.
3. **Your identity should not be built only on what you endured.**
   You are more than what you survived.
4. **Receiving help is not weakness—it's wisdom.**
   Independence learned through pain does not have to be permanent.
5. **Becoming begins when you allow yourself to want more without guilt.**
6. **You don't have to know who you'll be yet—just who you refuse to remain.**

## The To-Do List

If this chapter resonated with you, start here.

### 1. Redefine who you are

Finish this sentence in writing:

> "I am not just someone who survived. I am someone who is becoming ___________."

Say it out loud.

### 2. Identify the role you're ready to release

Ask yourself:

> "What identity have I been carrying that no longer fits my future?"

Examples:

- the strong one
- the fixer
- the struggler
- the one who always handles everything

Write it down—and give yourself permission to grow past it.

## 3. Practice receiving

This week, allow yourself to **receive** one thing without guilt:

- help
- rest
- encouragement
- opportunity

Notice how uncomfortable that feels—and stay with it.

## 4. Choose a new self-image

Write one sentence that describes the version of you that is emerging.

Example:

> "I am becoming a woman who chooses peace over proving."

Put it where you can see it daily.

### 5. Take one step toward your new identity

Ask:

> "What would the person I am becoming do differently this week?"

Then do that.

## Closing Reflection

You didn't change your life the day everything improved.
You changed it the day **you** did.

The moment you stopped defining yourself by survival...
you opened the door to transformation.

This chapter is proof that the real breakthrough wasn't external.

It was internal.

You didn't just survive your childhood.
You outgrew it.

And that is the beginning of everything.

# MEDICAL SCHOOL

## Reflection

This chapter shows the shift from asking, *Why did this happen to me?*
to asking, *How long am I willing to carry it?*

Many people survive their childhood only to spend adulthood reliving it—through resentment, anger, self-blame, or emotional walls built so high nothing new can get in. This chapter reveals the moment you realized that healing wasn't about changing the past.

It was about **releasing its power** over your present.

Forgiveness didn't come because everything felt resolved.
It came because you were tired of being heavy.

That's when growth moved from strength...
to **freedom**.

## The Lessons

1. **Forgiveness is not approval—it is release.**
   You can forgive without forgetting. You can forgive without returning.
2. **Unhealed anger keeps you tied to the past.**
   Healing cuts the cord.
3. **You don't owe anyone your peace—but you do owe it to yourself.**
4. **Closure doesn't always come from others.**
   Sometimes you give it to yourself.
5. **Healing begins when you stop waiting for an apology that may never come.**
6. **Freedom feels lighter than justice.**
   And lighter is better.

## The To-Do List

If this chapter touched something in you, begin here.

### 1. Name what you're still carrying

Finish this sentence in writing:

"I am still holding on to ___________."

Don't judge it. Just name it.

### 2. Redefine forgiveness

Write your own definition:

> "Forgiveness means __________."

Make sure it centers **your peace**, not their comfort.

### 3. Release one burden

Write down one memory, one resentment, or one regret you are ready to stop carrying.

Then write this underneath it:

> "I release this because my future deserves room."

### 4. Practice emotional boundaries

Ask yourself:

> "What would protecting my peace look like in this situation?"

Then act accordingly—without explanation.

### 5. Choose lightness

This week, choose **one moment** where you refuse to relive an old hurt.
Change the subject.
Leave the room.
Redirect your thoughts.

Freedom begins in small choices.

## Closing Reflection

You were never meant to carry what hurt you forever.

Pain is part of your story—
but it is not the narrator.

Forgiveness didn't erase your past.
It **unburdened your future**.

And in choosing freedom over fury,
peace over punishment,
healing over holding on...

you didn't lose anything.

You gained your life back.

# IMPOSTER SYNDROME

## Reflection

This chapter shows the shift from hoping someone else will change your life...
to realizing **you are the one who must choose it**.

For a long time, survival taught you to look outward:

- for rescue
- for permission
- for opportunity
- for someone to believe in you first

But this chapter reveals the moment you understood something quietly powerful:

No one was coming to rewrite your story.
You had to do it yourself.

Not all at once.
Not perfectly.
But intentionally.

This is the chapter where responsibility turns into **ownership** — not blame, not shame, but agency.

The moment you stopped asking, *Who will help me?* and started asking, *What can I build with what I have?*

That is the beginning of self-leadership.

## The Lessons

1. **Waiting feels safer than choosing — but it keeps you stuck.**
   Growth begins the moment you act without guarantees.
2. **You don't need permission to change your life.**
   You only need decision.
3. **Ownership is not blame — it is power.**
   Taking control doesn't mean you caused the pain. It means you control the healing.
4. **Small choices shape big futures.**
   You don't rise suddenly. You rise steadily.
5. **You don't need a perfect plan — you need movement.**

6. **Leadership of your life begins when excuses end.**

## The To-Do List

If this chapter stirred something in you, start here.

### 1. Write your ownership statement

Finish this sentence in writing:

> "I take responsibility for ____________."

Not your past.
Your **next step**.

### 2. Identify what you've been waiting for

Answer honestly:

> "I've been waiting for __________ to change before I change."

Now cross it out.
Write:

> "I choose to move anyway."

### 3. Choose one decision

This week, make **one clear decision** you've been avoiding.

Not ten.
Just one.

Examples:

- enrolling
- applying
- leaving
- saving
- starting

Momentum is born from decisions.

### 4. Replace waiting with action

Every time you think:

> "I'll do it someday..."

Replace it with:

> "I'll take one step today."

Then take it.

### 5. Write your leadership vow

Complete this sentence:

"From today forward, I lead my life by ____________."

Choose a value:

- courage
- honesty
- consistency
- self-respect
- faith

## Closing Reflection

You didn't change your life because someone finally helped you.

You changed your life because **you finally chose yourself.**

This chapter is proof that rescue is not always dramatic. Sometimes it looks like a quiet decision made in an ordinary moment.

A decision to stop waiting.
A decision to stop hoping someone else will fix it.
A decision to take your life back—one choice at a time.

And that is how real transformation begins.

Not when life saves you...
but when **you** do.

# DOCTOR

## Reflection

This chapter shows the shift from healing privately...
to living **intentionally**.

For a long time, your focus was on getting out, getting through, getting better. But this chapter reveals the deeper transformation—the moment you realized your story wasn't just something to recover from.

It was something to **rise from**.

This is where pain turns into purpose.
Where wounds turn into wisdom.
Where survival turns into **service**.

Not because you owed the world anything—
but because you finally understood how powerful your life really is.

This chapter shows the moment you stopped seeing your past as baggage...
and started seeing it as **foundation**.

## The Lessons

1. **Your story is not a liability — it is a leadership tool.**
   What you've survived gives you insight others can't learn in books.
2. **Healing is not the finish line — it is the starting point.**
   Once you heal, you get to choose how you live.
3. **You don't have to hide what made you — you can honor it.**
4. **Purpose grows where pain once lived.**
   What once hurt you can now help others.
5. **Your past doesn't define you — but it can empower you.**
6. **True growth means using your life to lift others, not just yourself.**

## The To-Do List

If this chapter moved you, begin here.

### 1. Name your influence

Finish this sentence in writing:

> "Because of what I've lived through, I can help others by ___________."

Don't minimize it. Your experience matters.

### 2. Reframe your past

Write one paragraph starting with:

> "My past prepared me to..."

Let yourself see your story through the lens of strength.

### 3. Choose your impact lane

Ask yourself:

> "Where do I feel called to make a difference?"

Examples:

- mentoring
- speaking
- writing
- parenting
- leadership
- community work

You don't need to do everything. Just choose one direction.

## 4. Take one purpose-driven step

This month, do **one thing** that uses your story for good:

- share it
- write it
- speak it
- live it more boldly

Purpose grows through action.

## 5. Write your legacy line

Complete this sentence:

> "When my life is remembered, I want it to be said that I ___________."

Let that guide your next season.

## Closing Reflection

You didn't survive your childhood just to move on from it.

You survived so you could **rise with it**.

Every tear taught you compassion.
Every loss taught you resilience.
Every moment you almost gave up taught you how to stay.

This chapter is not about the end of pain.

It is about the beginning of **purpose**.

And when you finally see your life not as something that happened to you...
but as something that is happening **through** you...

you step into the strongest version of yourself yet.

Not just healed.
Not just whole.

But **impactful**.

# BECOMING

## Reflection

This chapter shows what happens when you stop defining yourself by what you've lived through—and start imagining who you could become because of it. For a long time, your life trained you to be reactive. You learned how to respond to crisis, manage pain, and endure pressure. But becoming requires something different.

It requires **vision**.

This chapter captures the moment when you didn't yet have proof—but you allowed yourself to have **permission**. Permission to want more. Permission to dream without apology. Permission to imagine a life that didn't revolve around just getting through the day.

That moment is quiet, but it's revolutionary.

Because the day you stop seeing yourself only as a survivor... you begin to see yourself as a **builder**.

## The Lessons

1. **You don't need proof before you need permission.**
   Belief often comes before evidence.
2. **Survival builds strength. Becoming builds direction.**
   Endurance keeps you alive. Vision moves you forward.
3. **Your future begins when you allow yourself to want more without guilt.**
4. **New identity feels uncomfortable before it feels natural.**
   Growth always feels foreign at first.
5. **You don't become by accident. You become by decision.**
6. **The life you imagine is often the life calling you.**

## The To-Do List

If this chapter spoke to you, begin here.

### 1. Give yourself permission

Finish this sentence in writing:

> "I give myself permission to become _____."

Don't shrink it. Don't explain it. Just write it.

## 2. Identify the life you want

Answer honestly:

> "If I weren't afraid of failing, I would try __________."

That answer is your direction.

## 3. Name the old identity

Complete this sentence:

> "I am done living as __________."

Examples:

- the struggler
- the people-pleaser
- the one who settles
- the one who plays small

You can honor who you were and still outgrow them.

## 4. Choose one becoming action

This week, take **one action** that matches who you want to be—not who you've been.

Examples:

- enroll
- apply
- introduce yourself differently
- ask for help
- set a boundary
- invest in yourself

Becoming begins with behavior.

## 5. Write your vision line

Complete this sentence:

> "The person I am becoming is someone who ___________."

Read it every morning for seven days.

## Closing Reflection

You didn't wake up one day and suddenly become someone new.

You simply stopped accepting who you were forced to be.

That's how becoming begins.

Not with confidence.
Not with certainty.
But with **permission**.

Permission to want more.
Permission to imagine differently.
Permission to step into a life that once felt unreachable.

This chapter isn't about arrival.

It's about the first brave step into your future.

And once you take that step...
you never look at your life the same way again.

# SURVIVAL MODE

## Reflection

This chapter shows what happens after you decide you want more—when the reality of growth sets in. The dreams are no longer just ideas. They become effort. Discipline. Sacrifice. And suddenly, becoming doesn't feel inspiring anymore. It feels uncomfortable.

This is the stage where many people turn back.

Not because they can't grow...
but because growth asks them to leave who they've always been.

This chapter reveals the truth about transformation:

The hardest part of becoming isn't starting.
It's **staying**.

Staying when motivation fades.
Staying when old habits call you back.
Staying when progress feels slow and lonely.

This is where identity is truly rewritten—not in vision, but in **consistency**.

## The Lessons

1. **Excitement starts change. Discipline finishes it.**
   Feelings fade. Commitment carries you.
2. **Growth feels lonely before it feels rewarding.**
   Becoming often separates you from people and patterns that no longer fit.
3. **You don't outgrow your past without resistance.**
   Old habits fight to survive.
4. **Consistency matters more than confidence.**
   You don't need to feel ready—you need to keep showing up.
5. **Discomfort is not a sign you're failing.**
   It's often proof that you're changing.
6. **Staying is the real victory.**

## The To-Do List

If this chapter hit home, begin here.

### 1. Name what's getting harder

Finish this sentence honestly:

"Becoming feels difficult right now because ____________."

Don't judge the answer. Just tell the truth.

### 2. Identify your temptation to quit

Ask yourself:

"When things get hard, what do I usually run back to?"

Examples:

- old relationships
- old habits
- old excuses
- old comfort zones

Awareness weakens pull.

### 3. Choose consistency over intensity

Pick **one small habit** you will commit to for the next 30 days.

Not big.
Not dramatic.
Just steady.

Examples:

- ten minutes of reading
- walking daily
- saving $5
- writing one page
- saying no once a day

### 4. Rewrite your discomfort story

Finish this sentence:

> "This feels uncomfortable because I am ___________, not because I am failing."

Examples:

- growing
- changing
- healing
- leveling up

### 5. Make a staying promise

Write this and sign it:

> "I commit to staying in my growth even when it gets uncomfortable."

Put today's date under it.

## Closing Reflection

You didn't begin becoming because it was easy.
You began because staying the same hurt more.

This chapter is not about motivation.
It's about **maturity**.

The maturity to keep going when the excitement fades.
The maturity to choose growth over comfort.
The maturity to stay when leaving would be easier.

This is where real becoming happens.

Not in the moment you dreamed bigger...
but in the days you **refused to quit**.

And every day you stay...
you become stronger than you were before.

# LETTING GO

## Reflection

This chapter shows what happens when you begin to outgrow the life you once lived—while others are still living in it. When you change, not everyone celebrates. Some feel confused. Some feel threatened. Some feel left behind.

And suddenly, becoming isn't just personal anymore.
It's relational.

This is the stage where many people shrink back—not because they don't want to grow, but because they don't want to lose connection. They choose familiarity over authenticity. Belonging over becoming.

This chapter reveals the quiet courage it takes to choose yourself even when it costs comfort with others.

Because real growth always requires **new boundaries**.

Not walls.
But standards.

Not distance.
But clarity.

## The Lessons

1. **Growth changes who you walk with.**
   Not everyone is meant to go where you're going.
2. **You don't have to explain your becoming to everyone.**
   Some people understand through time, not words.
3. **Outgrowing others doesn't mean you're better.**
   It means you're different—and that's enough.
4. **Boundaries protect your future.**
   They are not punishments; they are promises to yourself.
5. **You can love people and still choose distance.**
   Both can be true.
6. **Becoming requires courage to stand alone before you stand supported.**

## The To-Do List

If this chapter felt close to home, begin here.

### 1. Identify who you've outgrown

Finish this sentence honestly:

"I feel myself growing away from __________
because __________."

This is clarity—not cruelty.

### 2. Define your new boundaries

Write down one boundary you need right now.

Examples:

- limiting certain conversations
- reducing access to your time
- saying no to draining relationships
- protecting your peace

### 3. Practice being misunderstood

Ask yourself:

> "Am I willing to be misunderstood in order to be authentic?"

Write your answer. Growth often requires yes.

## 4. Choose your inner circle

List the qualities you now need in the people closest to you.

Examples:

- honesty
- accountability
- encouragement
- respect
- growth-mindedness

Your environment shapes your future.

## 5. Take one boundary action

This week, take **one step** to protect your becoming.

Examples:

- decline an invitation
- limit a conversation
- speak your truth kindly

- step back from a draining dynamic

Boundaries build space for growth.

## Closing Reflection

You didn't change your life just to stay the same with everyone else.

You changed because you were becoming someone new.

And becoming someone new means choosing a life that fits who you are now—not who you used to be.

Some people will grow with you.
Some will grow away from you.

Both are part of the journey.

This chapter is not about loss.

It's about **alignment**.

And alignment always feels lonely before it feels right.

But when you choose yourself with clarity...
you make room for the people and the life that truly belong to you.

# PEACE

## Reflection

Peace is about the moment when **growth turns into leadership**.

Not leadership in a public sense.
Leadership in a personal one.

This chapter shows what happens when you stop becoming only for yourself—and start becoming for the life you want to build, the people you want to impact, and the future you want to leave behind.

At this stage, change is no longer new.
Healing is no longer fragile.
Growth is no longer accidental.

You are choosing your life on purpose.

This is where becoming shifts from:

- reaction to intention
- healing to direction
- survival to **stewardship**

You stop asking, *Who am I becoming?*
and start asking, *What am I building with who I've become?*

That question changes everything.

## The Lessons

1. **Growth matures into responsibility.**
   Becoming is not just about feeling better—it's about living better.
2. **Healing gives you clarity. Clarity gives you direction.**
   Direction turns change into legacy.
3. **Leadership begins at home—in your habits, your choices, your boundaries.**
4. **Your life is your loudest message.**
   People learn from what you live, not what you say.
5. **Becoming is not a phase—it's a posture.**
   A daily commitment to growth.
6. **The future you want is built by the decisions you make now.**

## The To-Do List

If this chapter feels like where you are right now, begin here.

### 1. Define what you're building

Finish this sentence:

> "With the person I am becoming, I want to build ___________."

Think long-term. Think legacy.

### 2. Identify your leadership lane

Ask yourself:

> "Where do I already influence others without realizing it?"

Examples:

- parenting
- work ethic
- relationships
- community
- faith
- consistency

That's your leadership starting point.

### 3. Choose one standard

Decide one **non-negotiable** for your life moving forward.

Examples:

- honesty in relationships
- respect in communication
- consistency in effort
- boundaries with time

Write it down. Live by it.

### 4. Create one legacy habit

Pick one habit that represents the life you want to build.

Examples:

- daily reflection
- weekly planning
- monthly goal setting
- regular gratitude
- intentional rest

Legacy grows from routines.

### 5. Write your future statement

Complete this sentence:

> "The life I am building now will be remembered for ___________."

Let that guide your decisions.

## Closing Reflection

You didn't survive everything you've been through just to heal quietly.

You survived so you could **live intentionally**.

This chapter is not about finally feeling okay.

It's about finally taking ownership of the life you are shaping.

Becoming is no longer something that happens to you.
It is something you **lead**.

And when you lead your life with clarity, courage, and consistency...
you don't just change yourself.

You change what's possible for everyone watching you.

# STILL HERE

## Reflection

*Still Here* is about the moment when survival becomes **meaning**.

Not success.
Not titles.
Not applause.

Meaning.

This chapter shows what happens when you stop measuring your life by what you escaped...
and start measuring it by what you **chose to stay for**.

So many people think strength is about never breaking.
But this chapter reveals the deeper truth:

Strength is staying.

Staying when it hurts.
Staying when you doubt yourself.
Staying when your past whispers that you're finished.

This chapter is the final shift—from becoming to **belonging**.
Belonging to your life.
Belonging to your future.
Belonging to yourself.

You didn't just survive your story.
You chose to remain in it—and reshape it.

That is what "still here" really means.

## The Lessons

1. **Survival gets you through. Presence gives you purpose.**
   You are no longer just enduring—you are living intentionally.
2. **You don't need to be fearless to be faithful to your life.**
   Staying is courage enough.
3. **Your life matters even without milestones.**
   Worth is not measured by achievements.

4. **Healing is learning to stay with yourself.**
   Not run. Not hide. Not disappear.
5. **Your presence is power.**
   Simply being here—fully—is impact.
6. **Almost is not failure. Almost is resilience.**

## The To-Do List

If this chapter feels like your truth, begin here.

### 1. Write your staying statement

Finish this sentence:

"I am still here because ___________."

Let it be honest. Let it be yours.

### 2. Acknowledge your survival

Write down three moments in your life when you could have given up—but didn't.

You don't need to justify them.
Just honor them.

## 3. Define what "being here" means now

Answer this:

"Being present in my life today looks like ___________."

Examples:

- resting when I'm tired
- speaking when I used to stay silent
- choosing peace over proving
- asking for help

## 4. Practice choosing life

This week, make one choice that affirms your life:

- say yes to something that brings peace
- say no to something that drains you
- slow down
- show up for yourself

Staying is built in small decisions.

### 5. Write your legacy line

Complete this sentence:

"If nothing else, my life will stand for ______________."

Let this be your compass.

## Closing Reflection

You are not here because life was easy.

You are here because you chose to **stay**.

When it would have been easier to disappear.
When it would have been easier to settle.
When it would have been easier to stop believing.

You stayed.

And that choice—quiet, steady, unseen—is the greatest victory of all.

Not unstoppable.
Not perfect.
Not finished.

Just **still here**.

And that...
is more powerful than any ending ever could be.

# ABOUT THE AUTHOR

Tiffanii Smith, MD is a first-generation physician whose life journey reflects resilience, determination, and purpose. Her path was shaped by obstacles that required strength, self-belief, and perseverance, ultimately leading her to a career dedicated to service and healing.

As the first in her family to enter medicine, Dr. Smith navigated unfamiliar territory with courage and focus, learning to trust the process even when the road ahead was unclear. The challenges she faced along the way became defining moments—lessons that built confidence, discipline, and a deep appreciation for growth.

Dr. Smith is the proud mother of three adult children and a loving grandmother to three grandchildren, whom she considers her greatest motivation and joy. Family remains central to her life, and she treasures time spent with her parents, siblings, extended family, and close friends who have supported her throughout every season.

Outside of medicine, Dr. Smith finds inspiration through traveling the world and experiencing new cultures. She has a lifelong love for classical music and Broadway productions, passions that bring balance, creativity, and reflection to her life. In her spare time, she values meaningful connection, laughter, and shared moments with those she loves most.

Through this memoir, Dr. Smith shares her story in hopes of encouraging others to push beyond limitations, trust their own resilience, and pursue goals that may once have felt out of reach. Her journey serves as a reminder that obstacles can become opportunities—and that purpose is often discovered by those willing to keep moving forward.

www.ingramcontent.com/pod-product-compliance
Lightning Source LLC
LaVergne TN
LVHW090401210926
848480LV00002B/418
* 9 7 9 8 9 0 2 7 1 0 4 2 4 *